Prepping for Survival in a Disaster

Be Tougher than the Disasters

Prepping and Survival Series

Sneha Agrawal

Mendon Cottage Books

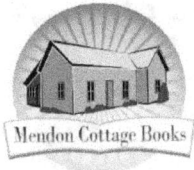

JD-Biz Publishing

Disclaimer

The information is this book is provided for informational purposes only. It is not intended to be used and medical advice or a substitute for proper medical treatment by a qualified health care provider. The information is believed to be accurate as presented based on research by the author.

The contents have not been evaluated by the U.S. Food and Drug Administration or any other Government or Health Organization and the contents in this book are not to be used to treat cure or prevent disease.

The author or publisher is not responsible for the use or safety of any diet, procedure or treatment mentioned in this book. The author or publisher is not responsible for errors or omissions that may exist.

Warning

The Book is for informational purposes only and before taking on any diet, treatment or medical procedure, it is recommended to consult with your primary health care provider.

Our books are available at

1. Amazon.com
2. Barnes and Noble
3. Itunes
4. Kobo
5. Smashwords
6. Google Play Books

Table of Contents

Introduction

Disasters just happen; they do not send signals before happening, and one must be prepared to combat any such situations in life. Disaster management is basically the self-preparedness before a disaster, at the time of the disaster and post disaster. Being prepared for the worst does not necessarily mean you will avoid worst, but it can definitely mitigate the effects of the worst.

Disasters can be caused naturally, and can be planned to bring some harm to a specific person or to a group of people. Whatever the case may be, it still brings a lot of pain and suffering along with it. This is why it is important that we try our best to avoid any kind of disasters from affecting our own lives.

Disasters have certain features, and one must be prepared according to the type of the disaster. The features are listed below:

-Duration (short term vs. long term)

Some kinds of disasters happen for a short interval of time and it takes less time to bring our lives back on track, whereas some of them take a lot of time to resolve. A classic example for the first scenario can be a local riot and the second one can be nuclear radiation out of a chemical blast.

-Scale (affecting individual or masses)

There are a few situations that are very personal in nature, like your career getting sabotaged, or your water heater breaking. Then there are other circumstances like terrorist attacks, floods and etc., which inflict pain among a huge mass.

-Recovery Time (Days/ Months/ Years)

Situations like local theft or protests get under control within few days, but there are situations like nuclear radiation that leaves their effects for years to come.

Chapter 1 – Disaster Management Cycle

Disaster management is a combination of sequential steps, taken in order, to minimize the damage caused because of some disastrous events. It is a whole cycle and the steps are explained below.

Prevention/Mitigation

There are accidents, which cannot be avoided, because we usually do not have any kind of control over such untimely events, but if possible, we should try and avoid the accident. We often come across a cliché; "It is not actually the problem but our attitude towards the problem, which determines the damaging effect it will have on us". Though it is a cliché, it holds very true in every kind of scenario. This is the reason that one should display a few characteristics like vigilance, mental strength, logical thinking mind, and a brave heart, in any disastrous situation. Being strong on all these fronts plays an important role in preventing any kind of disaster. A classic example of preventing disaster, would be avoiding any kind of theft in your house, by keeping proper safety measures in effect.

Preparedness

Despite remaining vigilant, there are situations in life, in which we unknowingly get trapped. Disastrous events are bound to happen and one should have some backup plans to overcome any kind of mishaps. Having a backup plan for survival is known as being prepared to fight in any kind of situation and not giving up. Again, taking the previous example of theft; though we do not want a thief to enter our house, we should always anticipate such an event. If a thief enters the house, we should not panic, and should be prepared to fight back. We should have the emergency helpline number on our speed dial, so that it can be used in such situations.

On site action

This basically says about how we fight back with the disaster, in any kind of situation. This tells a lot about our own characteristics; whether we give up in a tough situation or we decide to fight back and turn the situation in our favor. When the thief enters our house, then we have two options in front of us. Either we keep quiet and let him take away all our things we work hard for, or we fight to save the things that are precious to us. If we decide to fight back then we should know how to call for help in such a situation, and trap the thief until help comes.

Surviving post-affects

It may so happen that the attack we face leaves certain after-effects on us. We should be able to survive the post- effects of any kind of disaster. Let us take a hypothetical example that our house is situated within a vicinity of a chemical factory and one fine day we witness a chemical blast in the factory. Even if the blast is not life threatening, it will leave some black residue in the air for quite some time, and will affect our breathing. The damage has been done and we should then know how to behave at such times. We should always cover our mouth with a face mask, so that we do not inhale the polluted air, because of the chemical blast that happened.

We do not work in isolation in this world, and there is a multitude of things that we are surrounded with. We are surrounded with known and unknown people, manmade objects and of course nature. Any of these factors can bring in any kind of disastrous situation, into our personal lives. Further in this book, we will get a quick snapshot of the kinds of disasters we face in our day to day life.

Chapter 2 – Kinds of Disasters

Terrorism

The world is not free of anti-social elements. There are the people who do not love their own lives and are keen on making other's lives miserable. If we look in retrospect, then we will find that there have been innumerable instances that terrorist activities have left us in anarchy, and have made our lives miserable. The main intention of a terrorist is to spread fear among the common public and the government of the country. When there is fear in the hearts of people, every aspect of that particular state is affected; right from economy to religion. The terrorist activities are divided into a few sub categories

Terrorist activities at borders: These activities are more prevalent in Middle Eastern and Asian countries.

Hijack and attack: One classic example of this kind of terrorist activity is the 9/11 incident that happened in America, wherein a few terrorists hijacked several planes and crashed it into the twin towers and multiple other places. It has been over a decade since that the incident took place, but it still instills that fear in the minds of people who recall the happenings of that day.

Bombing: This is one of the easiest kinds of terrorist activities, where the terrorists plant a few bombs in a particular city, at a crowded place, and attack innocent lives.

Open terrorist activity: This is a rare event where the terrorists actually show up themselves in the open. They attack closed and crowded structures like malls, schools, hospitals, etc., and take hostages. They demand for fulfillment of their imposition, in lieu of freeing the hostages.

Sabotage

When a person is deliberately destroying the public or private property, to gain some political or military advantage, then that kind of event is known as sabotage. This can even become very personal in nature, as in amongst competitive peers, who are fighting to be promoted. To win over the situation, a particular employee can sabotage the promotional options of another employee.

Natural disaster

Mother earth has her own ways of taking the revenge from her residents in forms of various kinds of disasters. If we broadly categorize them then we see that natural disasters basically happen on land and through water. A few examples of such disasters are landslides, earthquakes, volcano eruption, Tsunamis, floods, pandemic influenzas and many more.

Public disorder

This kind of disaster does not affect a large group of people, but is highly damaging for the people who get involved in such instances. A few examples could be theft locally, an accident on the road, sexual harassment, and many others. They are short lived, but leave their scars for a long time to come.

Industrial accidents

These are disasters happening because of man-made mishandlings. A few examples of these are biological accidents in labs, furnace explosions in some industry, fire explosions at a factory site, blackouts, and many more.

Technological mishaps

With the fast development of technology and the ease that it provides, we have become very much dependent upon the gadgets like laptops, cell phones, etc. We also rely on technology driven transactions like e-mails, bank transfers, and many more. Now, imagine a situation where your laptop or your cell phone gets hacked or someone breaks all your firewall protection to get your financial secrets. Such events are categorized under disasters driven by technological advancements.

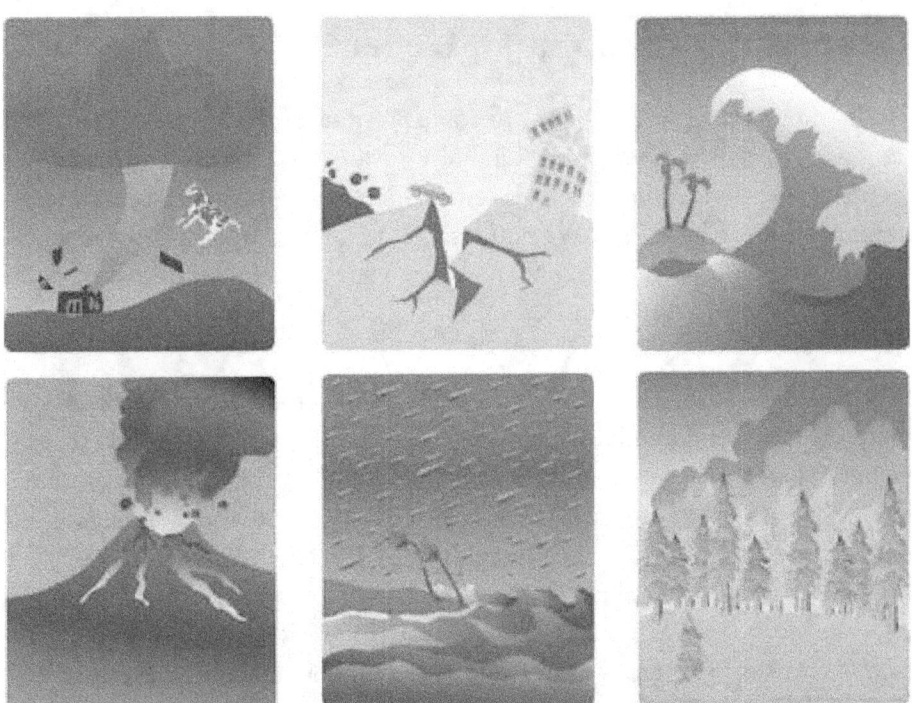

Collage depicting all Kinds of Disasters

Chapter 3 – Prepping in General

Further in this book, we will look at some pre-requisites, which are important for you to combat any kind of disaster successfully. The pre-requisites are divided into general steps, which are applicable to almost all kinds of disaster situations. We will also get to know the specific steps that one should take in order to avoid or sustain a specific kind of disaster.

Food supplies

Food is the basic requirement of any person, and is the energy source of our body. At times of natural disasters like flood, storms, etc., we usually face power cuts for weeks to come and we also cannot use solar heaters to cook our food. This is one reason that we should always have a stock of some kind of packed food, which can be sustained for a few days to come. Any kind of natural disaster stays for days and the government starts relief camps once the storm has passed away. They throw food packets on our terrace to avail us proper food, and we should remain vigilant enough to get our share of food packets.

Water storage

Nowadays we are all used to drinking filtered water and supply water that is available readily in our houses. At the time of a disaster, this water supply is cut for some time because of some disruptions. We should have some kind of backup for the water supply. We need to know how to harness the rain water and use it for drinking purposes. If you need to evacuate the place, you should still have some water storage to sustain you for a day or two.

Development of Basement

If you have your own house, and if it is suitable, then one should always look for creating a basement area within the house. This basement should be deep down enough, so that if some kind of biological disaster occurs, you can hide yourself from its dangers in your basement area. The basement should be radiation proof and it should contain essential supplies like packed food, water, clothes, sleeping bags, etc. so that you can stay there for a few weeks' time.

Precious items

It is always a good idea to keep all your precious belongings in a locker, far from your own place. The list of precious goods includes jewelry, will papers, power of attorney, and any other valuable items in your life.

Guide book

Knowledge about anything is good, and when it is about maintaining your safety, then, it becomes all the more important to remain informed. In order to remain prepared, one should always have a survival guide book handy, so that you can refer back to such a guide at the time of a crisis and take necessary actions.

Local Map and Compass

If you are supposed to evacuate your house for any reason, then you should have a local map of the area, so that you know that where you can go and which road will lead to which place. We should also carry a compass along with the map, because maps will lead us to the places and the compass will show us the direction to reach that place.

Survival kit

One should always keep an updated survival kit in place. If you are ever supposed to evacuate your house for safety reasons, you need to take this also. This kit should have some essential items like canned food, sleeping bags, guide book, torch, batteries, first-aid kit, and documents proving your identity, radio, knife and a set of clothes. It is also a good idea to carry a source of entertainment like an I-pod, fictional book or anything else that keeps you engaged and takes your mind from the disaster struck.

Other essentials

When we do not know where we are heading to, during evacuation process, then we must have some kind of food supply and a medium to cook food. Yes, we do have an option for that, in the form of portable solar cookers. They are easy to carry and can be used to cook the food in an emergency. We should also carry a bottle of honey. This can be used for multiple purposes. It can be used to heal a wound and can also be used as food. Honey does not degrade fast, and has lot of potential to supply you with adequate energy.

Proper attire

If you are supposed to leave your house, then you should know about your dress code. It is advised to wear something comfortable and easy to carry. One should also wear some comfortable shoes so that if you are supposed to walk a lot, your legs do not hurt. This attire should always be kept handy, so that at the time of emergency evacuation you can dress in a very short time.

After looking at some general steps, now we will look at some specific situations and the ways of remaining prepared to overcome the disastrous situation.

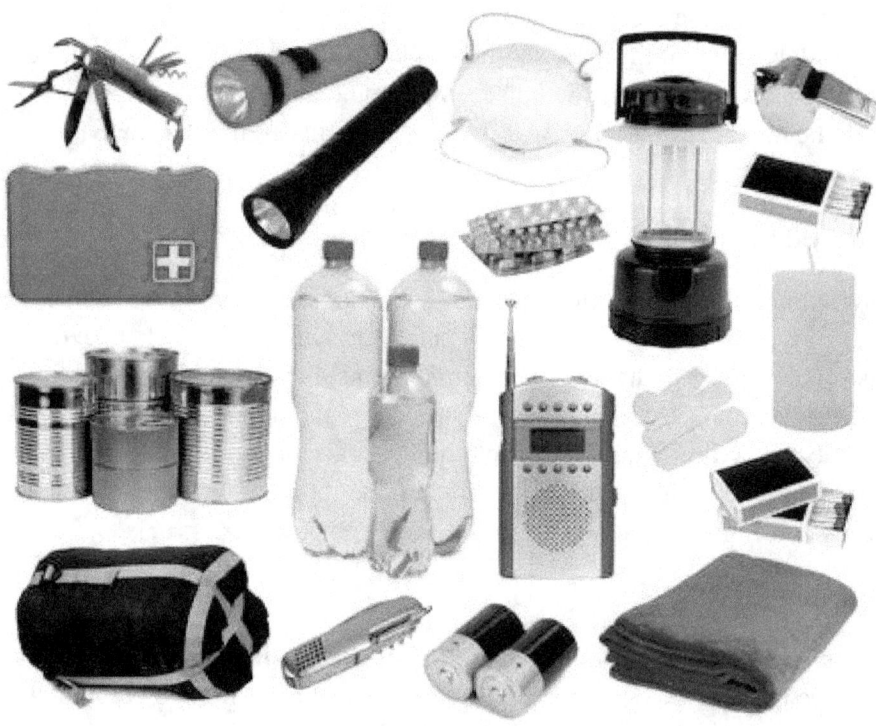

Disaster Management Survival Kit

Chapter 4 – Survival during a Terrorist Attacks

In this era of fast development, we also develop the negative activities around us really fast. One such activity is a terrorist attack, in a different form than mentioned above in the book. Terrorists neither play by rules, nor show sympathy for anyone in specific. When they attack, it brings in mass destruction and terror. Nevertheless, there are measures which can be taken, so that the damaging effects of the attack are mitigated. At the time of a terrorist attack, we could be either asked to stay back in our respective places or we might be asked to evacuate our place for safety reasons. We should be prepared for both the scenarios. We must listen to the radio and the latest announcements from the government, and get prepared accordingly. We must also listen to the local authorities diligently and follow the instructions given by them. If time permits, then we must try to reach out to our near and dear ones through some medium. At the time of an attack, usually the phone traffic gets overloaded and we might not be able to reach to the other person via telephone; e-mail on the other hand, does help. A point of contact should be known in advance, so that all the people stuck somewhere are able to contact that single point of contact. This contact should be someone away from the city under attack.

If we are supposed to evacuate our place, then we will be guided by the local authority about the place we are supposed to reach, and it is our duty to follow their commands. In such situations, they are the charge in command, and they know best about our safe whereabouts. We should form a group and then head to the place suggested to us. We should carry our supply kit and also take care of the elders, who need our help.

When the attack is happening all over the city, then the safest place to hide is our own house. We must at first check on children present at school and then ensure that they are under the guidance of a responsible authority. Getting them dropped at home might not be a good idea, as we do not know about the situation outside the school premise. We must have the plastic sheets and duct tape handy, so that we can cover all the windows with them. We should not rush to open the door, if we get a knock on the door. We must first ensure about the whereabouts of the person at the door by looking at the peephole and key hole, identify him/her, and then only open the door. If we are asked to switch off the natural gas supply, then we must have back-up plans like solar cookers, to be able to cook food for ourselves. The most important thing is to remain calm at such times, and think straight. A lot can be solved if we are able to maintain our calm, and a lot can be lost if we lose our temper.

Chapter 5 – Survival during a Natural Disaster

Natural disasters are very unpredictable in nature, and sometimes they give us no time to prepare for the danger. However, we can remain prepared for such disasters on the basis of our geographical locations. For example, if we reside near a beach area, then we should accordingly be prepared for floods, heavy rainfall and fast moving winds. On the other hand, if we stay in an earth-quake prone area, then we should be prepared accordingly by tying down furniture and making sure that heavy items stay close to the floor. There are a few specific techniques which can help us during such calamities.

If we take an example of the most earth quake prone country, Japan, then we will know that the locales are used to such situations on a daily basis; we can actually learn from them, on the ways of survival at times of earthquakes. At first, if we get that feeling of vibration of the earth, then we must anticipate that it can be because of the tectonic movements below earth. If we are stuck in a house or a huge building, then we should leave the premise as soon as possible, and move out to an open field. We should locate such a spot, which is isolated from any tall buildings nearby, and do not have any other big structures around us. In the case of earthquakes, those buildings might fall because of the vibrations and they might hurt us.

If we are stuck in a building and we are not able to move out of the building, then we must protect ourselves by remaining inside the building itself. We must look around ourselves and locate a place to hide. The selection of the place is very important here because it should have a specific design. There has to be a division which is formed by the long shaft and a central support beneath it, for example a table. Now, when the earthquake strikes, then the table top will break and fall either to our left or to our right, and other things that fall from the top, will either slide down towards our left or right. They will not fall directly on our head and will save us from the danger.

There is another kind of natural disaster that we face during rainy season, and that is lightning strikes. At first we should ensure that we are living in a house where proper grounding has been done. This will ensure that, if any current is flowing within the house, will go straight to the ground level in the earth. At the time of a lightning strike, we need to ensure that none of the electrical appliances like freezers, cable wires, laptops, kitchen appliances, and any other such devices have shorted out. When the lightning strikes, it brings in a high voltage of electricity with it. If that current somehow gets routed to our electrical appliances, then it might cause serious damage, and in the worst case scenario, the appliance might even burst. So, it is best to unplug them and cut back all the power supply to the house. If at all we have a basement area in our house, then we must shift to that area for some time, and be around the wooden base.

There are other events, like floods and hurricanes, which can only be avoided if we remain vigilant, get the signals from nature, and vacate the place before the storm has struck the city. Even if we are not able to vacate the storm hit area in time, we can save ourselves by following a few rules. If we look at the past statistics, then the most disastrous hurricane, Katrina, took numerous lives because people were not prepared to combat such a situation, and had a lack of disaster management knowledge. All the flood water entered people's houses and made them immovable. People got trapped inside their houses and could not move out, to save their lives.

At the times of a flood or a hurricane, it is best that we relocate ourselves to the top most story of the building, wherein water logging would become tough. We should also have a few sharp and heavy objects, like an axe, to help break the windows and doors, and let the water flow outside. This method will save us from the situation of water logging. At the times of a flood and a hurricane, usually the water supply gets disturbed, so we should take necessary measures to save the water stored in the tanks. We should stop flushing the toilet, and store all the halt water in the pipes in our water tanks.

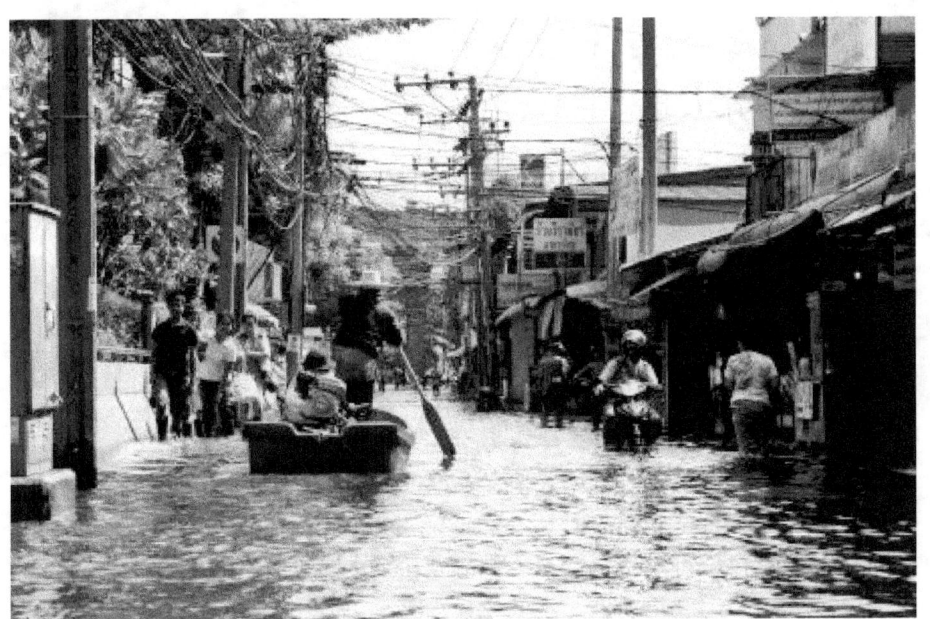

Chapter 6 – Survival during Chemical or Manmade Disasters

Apart from the natural disasters, there are calamities which we unknowingly bring on ourselves which are given the name of manmade calamity. Usually we see such disasters happen at a factory site or a research center, because of an incorrect experiment or some kind of mishandling. If we live within the area that is affected by some kind of nuclear radiation, then we must immediately vacate that area. We cannot stop nuclear radiation from entering our houses, even if we hide behind iron walls. It will affect us in any case and thus the best way to get away from them is by relocating to a safe area for days, weeks, or months to come. Before we leave the area, we should get checked out to ensure that we are not already affected by the radiation, and take necessary anti-dotes if required.

Chemical blasts affect us in two ways. At first it pollutes the air around us and the waste chemicals are absorbed deep down into the earth and infect the water beds. Immediately after the chemical hazard, we should take extra care in purifying the water we drink. We should always drink the purified water and if possible drink the mineral water only. Mineral water is produced at a far away, non-infected place and is safe for drinking.

Chapter 7 – Surviving Disasters of Sabotage

Apart from all the natural disasters, there are situations which are created intentionally to affect someone negatively. This is done to gain any kind of personal advantage over a situation or a thing. One classic example of this kind of situation is undergoing a sabotage situation in the professional environment that you are in. You might be a successful employee, the most suitable prospect of getting a promotion, and most liked by all your bosses. These traits are usually not liked by your co-workers and they try and damage your reputation and jeopardize your option of getting promoted. They can actually damage all your career goals and success plans in life. It is totally your responsibility to take care of yourself at such situations.

You must never share your computer, e-mail, official mail, and etc. passwords, with any of your colleagues, even if he is the most trustworthy peer of yours. You never know, who might backstab you. You should also never disclose all your trade secrets to the people whom you are working with, and also remain vigilant so that nobody takes the credit of your own work. Your personal computers have a lot of information and you must keep the password secret and do not write them on a piece of paper or anywhere else. Never share your finished project with someone else, otherwise they might steal your work and get all the credit for your good work. Even if you have been ditched, tell it to your boss, because no matter what your boss knows about you, they might come to your rescue. At last, do not show blind trust to the people whom you are working with, because you might have an enemy disguised as a best friend, at your workplace.

There are a few damages which are caused to one specific gender of our society; the female section of the society. Even teasing is a kind of disaster which is faced by all sections of society, and by all the classes. This can even turn into a serious disastrous situation for the woman, in the form of sexual harassment. Sexual harassment is a personal disaster which spoils the life of a female and thus it is a female's whole and sole responsibility to avoid any such situations in life.

They should always remain vigilant and should always keep a close eye on the events happening around them. For example, if they are in a shopping complex and buying an outfit, then before entering into the changing room they should ensure that their phone has proper signals within the dressing room. If the signals are not proper, this means that there is a hidden camera placed in that changing room, which might capture unwanted pictures of the female. While travelling alone, they should always keep a bottle of pepper spray in their purse, so that they can fight with the anti-social elements. The women should also know about all the help line numbers which are dedicated for women, and are ready to help in just one call.

Chapter 8 – Surviving a Disaster of Public Disorder

There are situations in life when we come across disasters like community theft, and local public disorder. It affects us and the neighborhood we stay in. An example of this is community theft, wherein a series of houses have been looted and the thief is not caught. There are a few major steps we need to take for avoiding a theft happening at our house and locality. We should postpone all our travelling plans for a future date if possible, because thieves attack the houses when they are empty; if the travelling cannot be avoided, then we should get a trusted person to take care of our house in our absence. We should also form a disaster management community with some representatives of our community and hire a private detective, who can catch hold of the thief. Whether we stay in apartments, or houses, we can get a security camera fixed at various angles within the society, so that we are able to track all the things happening in the premise of the society. This vigilance will also help us in knowing about the thief and can help us in overcoming any major disasters.

We even face situations like communal riots, which usually are done to fulfill certain political ambitions, but hamper the life of the common mass. We should remain prepared at all times for such distress in the society, because these are the times when anti-social elements take advantage of riots and damage other's property. At times of communal riots, we should refrain ourselves from moving out of our houses. Communal riots happen at a specific location in a city, so if we need to pick up children from school, we should not go out and do it; rather we should get them picked up by a friend or family member of ours that stays in an area that not disturbed by the riot. This is best for our own safety and our children's safety. We should always keep the police helpline number handy, so that if the need should arise, we are able to call for police help immediately.

We should even take care of our personal belongings during such times. We should park our cars and other vehicles properly in the garage, so that the anti-social elements are not able to damage any of our personal properties. We may not be able to move out of our houses, for a few days altogether, because of a red alert in such disturbed areas. So in such situations, we should keep ourselves informed about the latest happenings on the radio, and maintain our calm.

Chapter 9 – Surviving Disasters of Technical Mishaps

Today all our world has shrunk to online portals and a majority of our work is done online itself. We get online jobs, get paid online, and we place online orders to use the earned money for our daily necessities. Now, think of a scenario where your bank account gets hacked and all your earnings get transferred to some other account. Nothing can be more disastrous than having lost all your money because of an online robber. There are ways, however, to avoid such situations in life. At first, whatever online payments we do, should be done from our personal laptops/ desktops or cell phones. These transactions are supposed to be done with good internet connectivity, and from the instruments that have been protected with the latest firewalls.

Usually the hacker builds a virus and sends the links to us via an e-mail. We should refrain ourselves from opening e-mails from any unknown e-mail ids, as they might contain a virus. While doing any kind of banking transactions, we should ensure that the URL we are using starts from https:/ and not http:/. The later one is usually a dummy site created by hackers to get your passwords.

Let us understand the situation in detail, with an example. Let us say that you have an account with xyz bank, and you have opened the home page to that bank, to make some online transfers. Now, once you enter all the required details and the password and press enter, you find that your computer show a "page not found" screen. This might be because you have entered your bank details in some dummy site. Now, as soon as you face this issue, just call up your bank and tell them to stop any kind of transfers from your account, and lock your account until further instructions from you. Once you have changed all your passwords and etc., you can again activate your account. This will save your money from being stolen online.

Once you have made any kind of payments online, then you get a message in your number confirming the payment. Check the messages of your bank diligently, as all the messages might not be a promotional message and can actually save your money from getting looted.

Conclusion

Life is very unpredictable, and we never know what is in store for us, in the future. The future might be bright, but it can also be disastrous. Nevertheless, it totally depends upon us, how we take a particular situation. Even if we enter into any kind of disastrous situation, we should think straight and keep calm. If we are able to think straight, even at times of crisis, we will be able to find a solution to the problem in our hand. We should also be prepared for any kind of crisis situations occurring in our life, so that we know how to handle a particular situation. In this book we got to know about various kinds of disaster, how they strike, and the ways of combating such disastrous situations. Now that you have read the book, you are more prepared to take on the disastrous situations of our life and make the most out of this beautiful life. We actually get life just once, and we should not lose it just because of our unwillingness to be prepared for the worst.

Author Bio

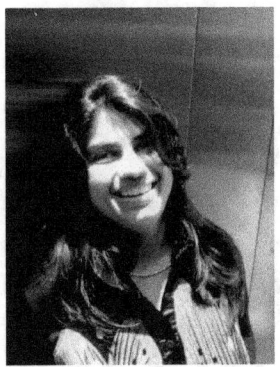

Books are a great medium of sharing one's own experiences with the outer world, and enhancing the knowledge of the readers. With this same purpose, I, Sneha Agrawal share this write-up with my readers.

I am an MBA graduate from a top notch Business School of India, and have done specialization in marketing and finance stream. I also hold some work experience as a team leader, for one of the known Indian IT companies.

To live a successful life, one should always have the answers of a few questions, at any point in time and they are what, how and when; and I live my life in search of these answers.

Check out some of the other JD-Biz Publishing books

Gardening Series on Amazon

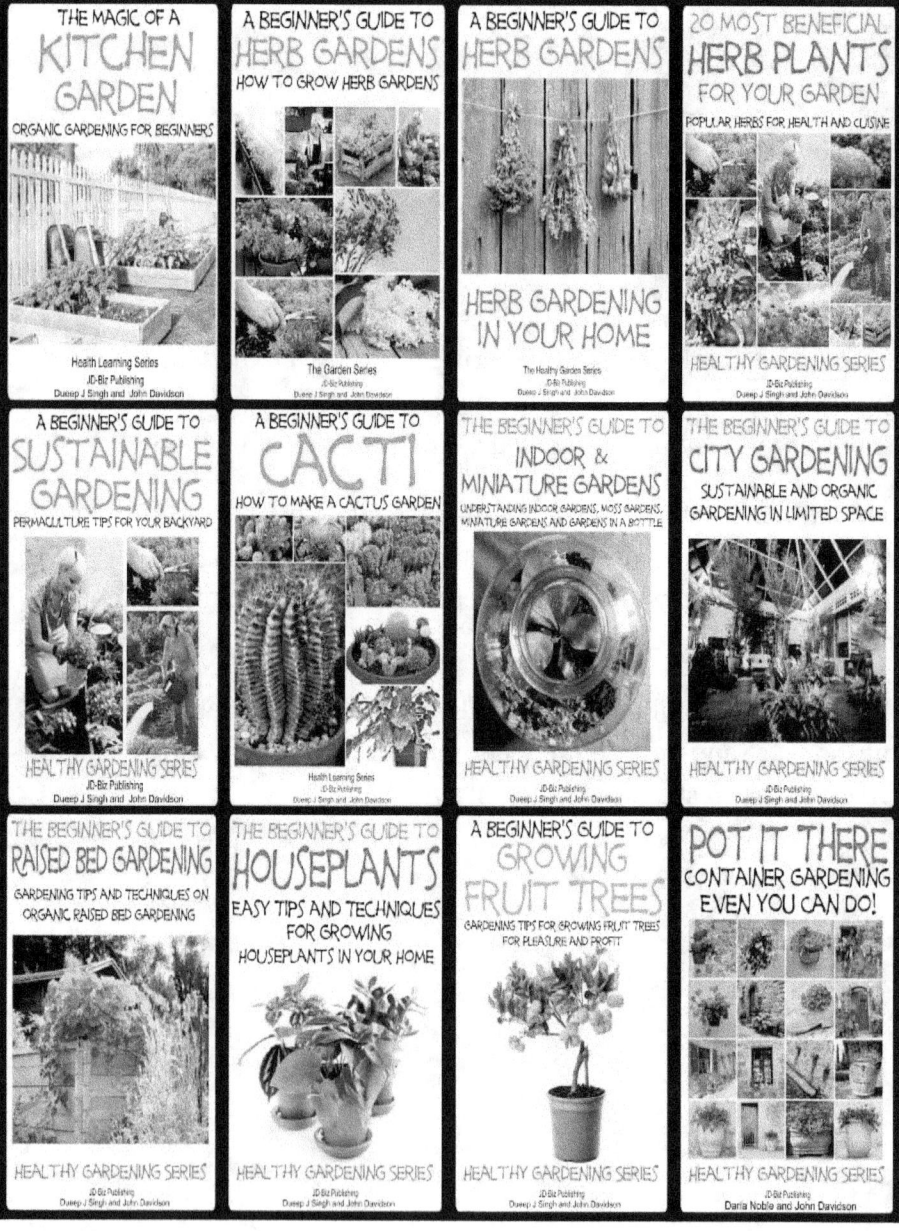

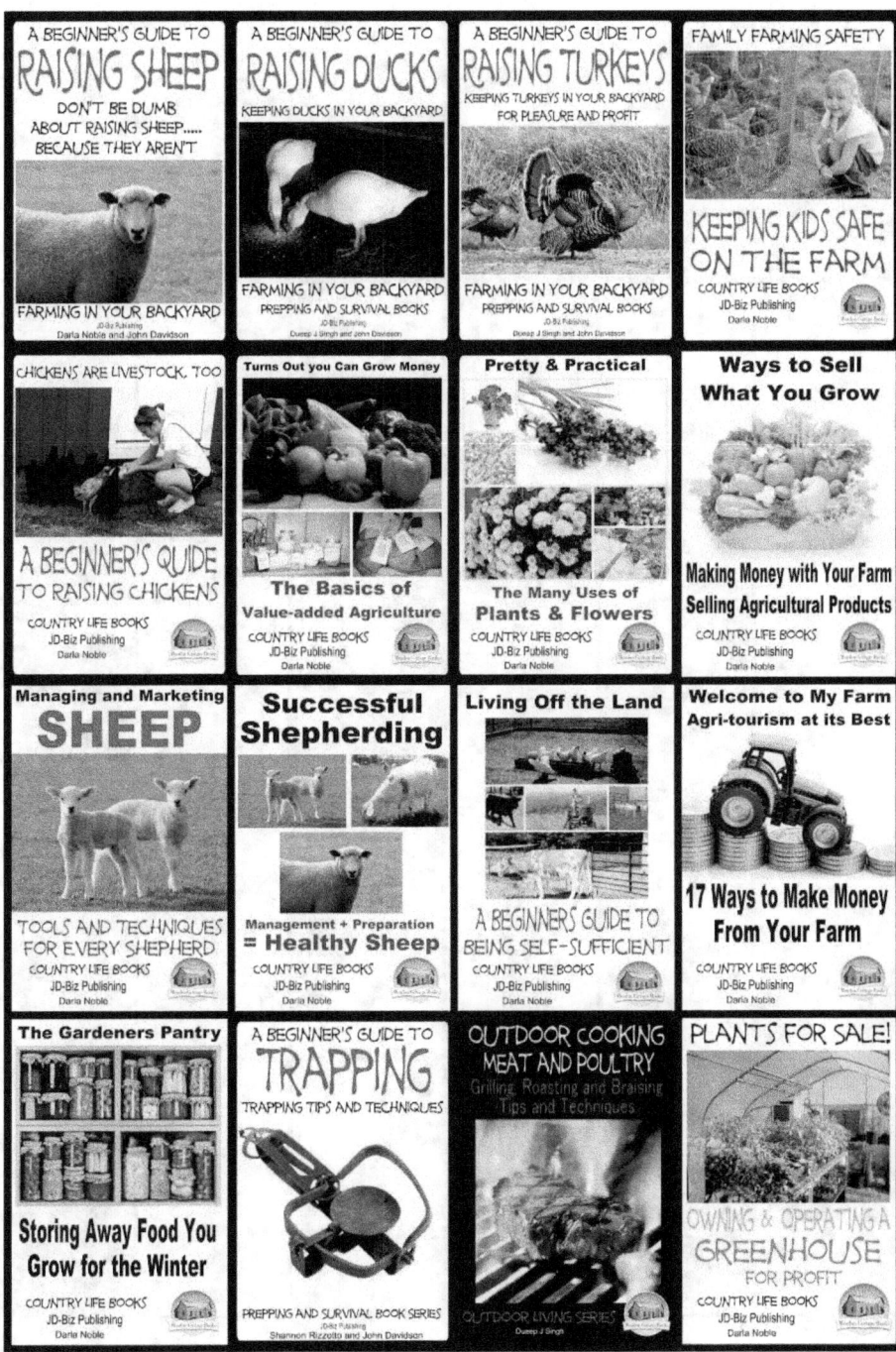

Health Learning Series

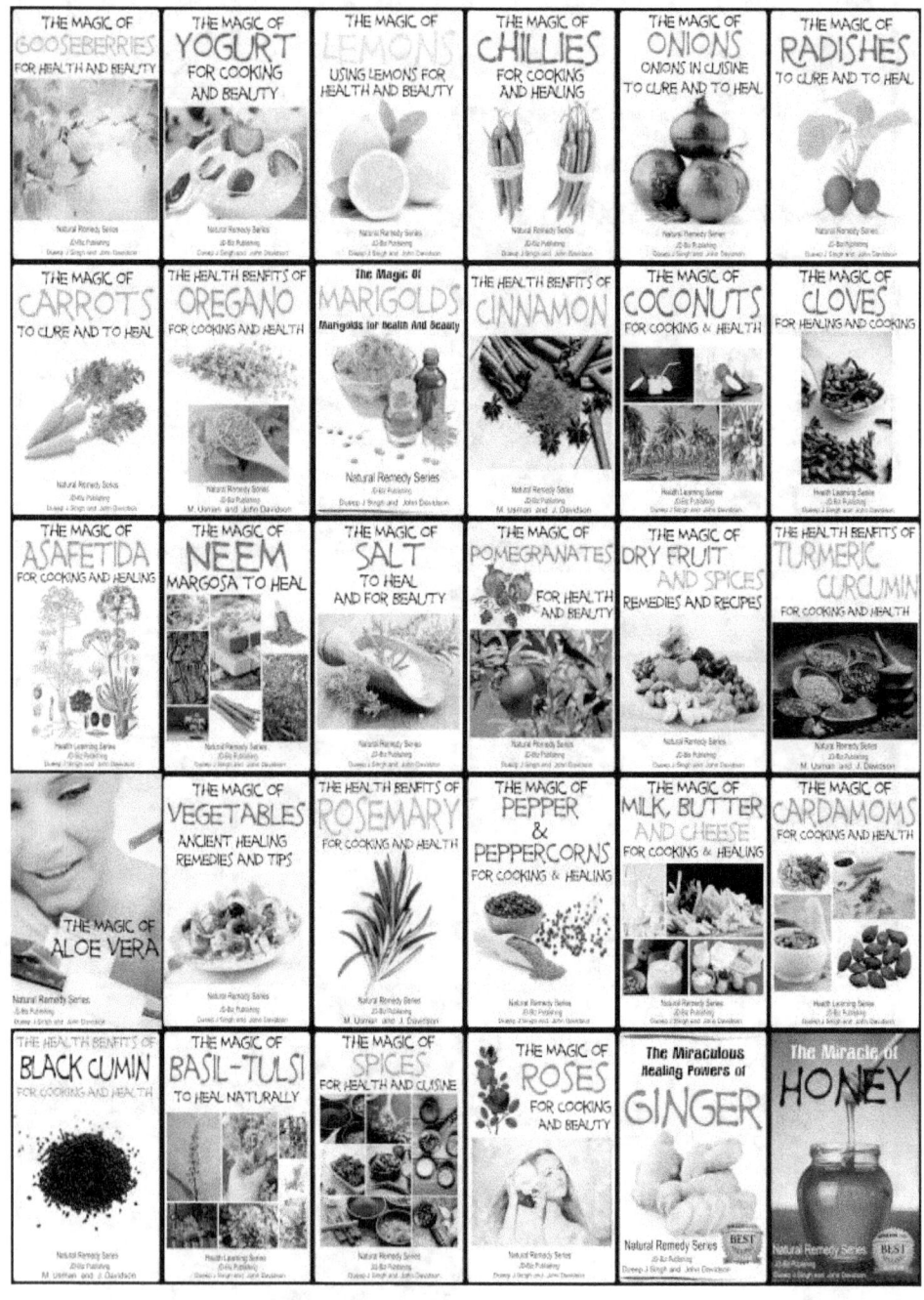

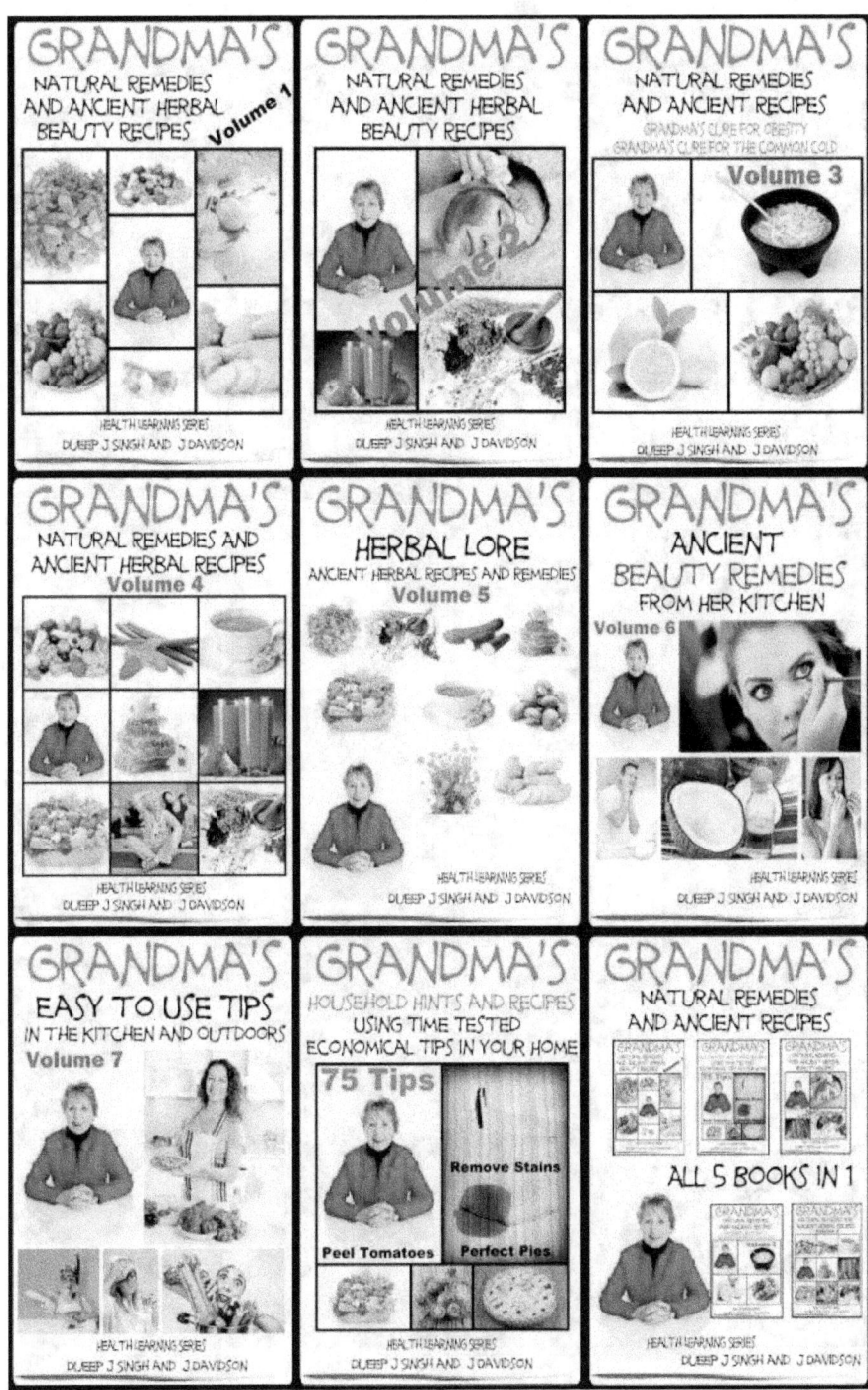

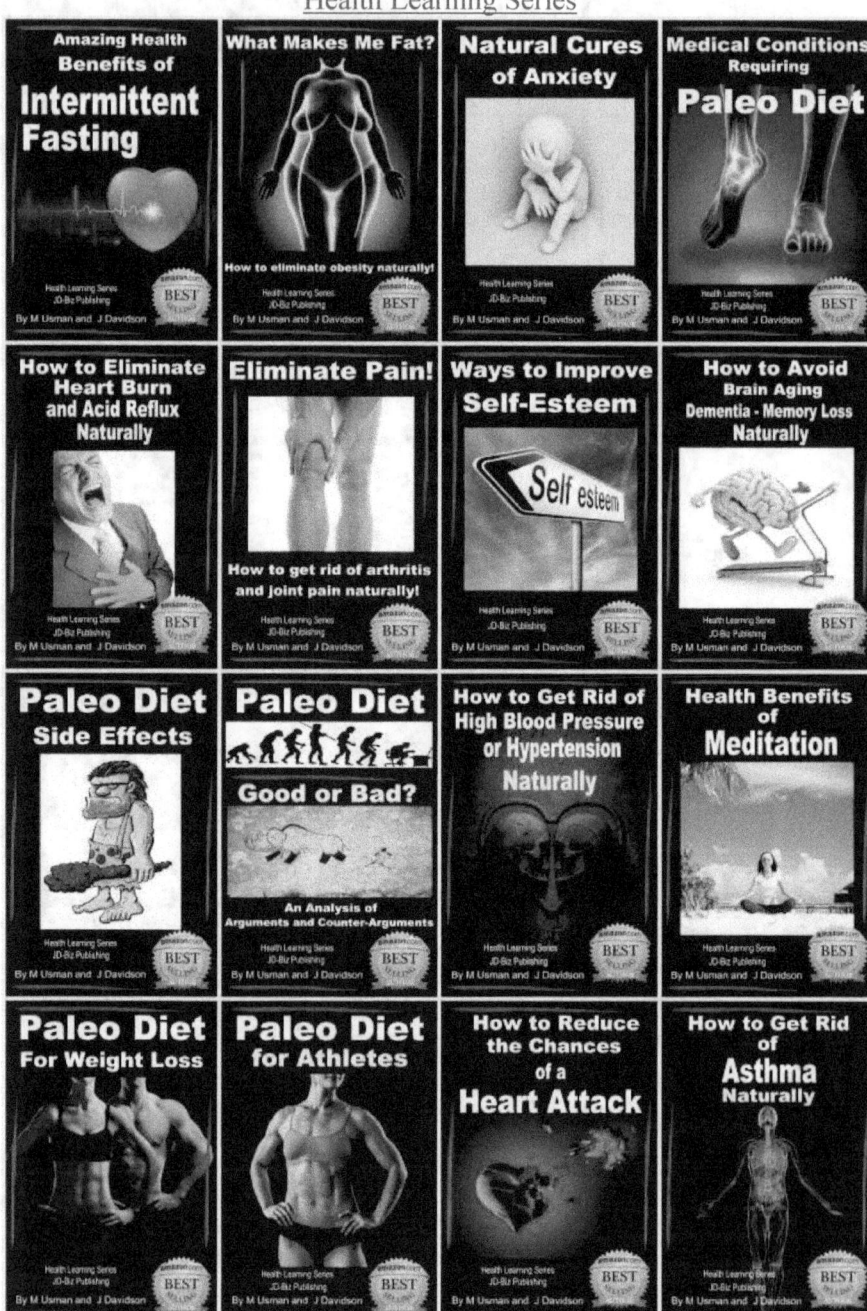

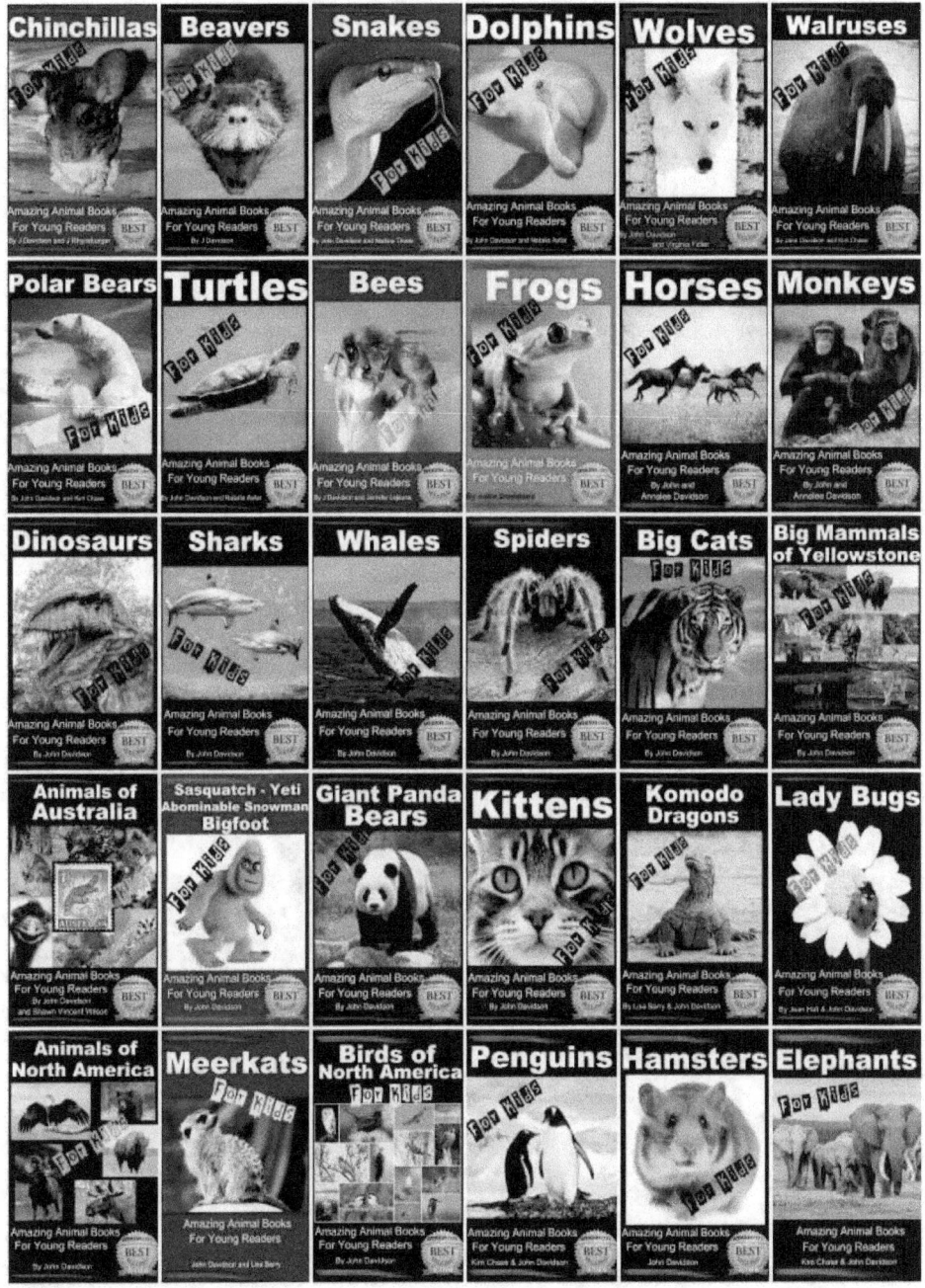

Learn To Draw Series

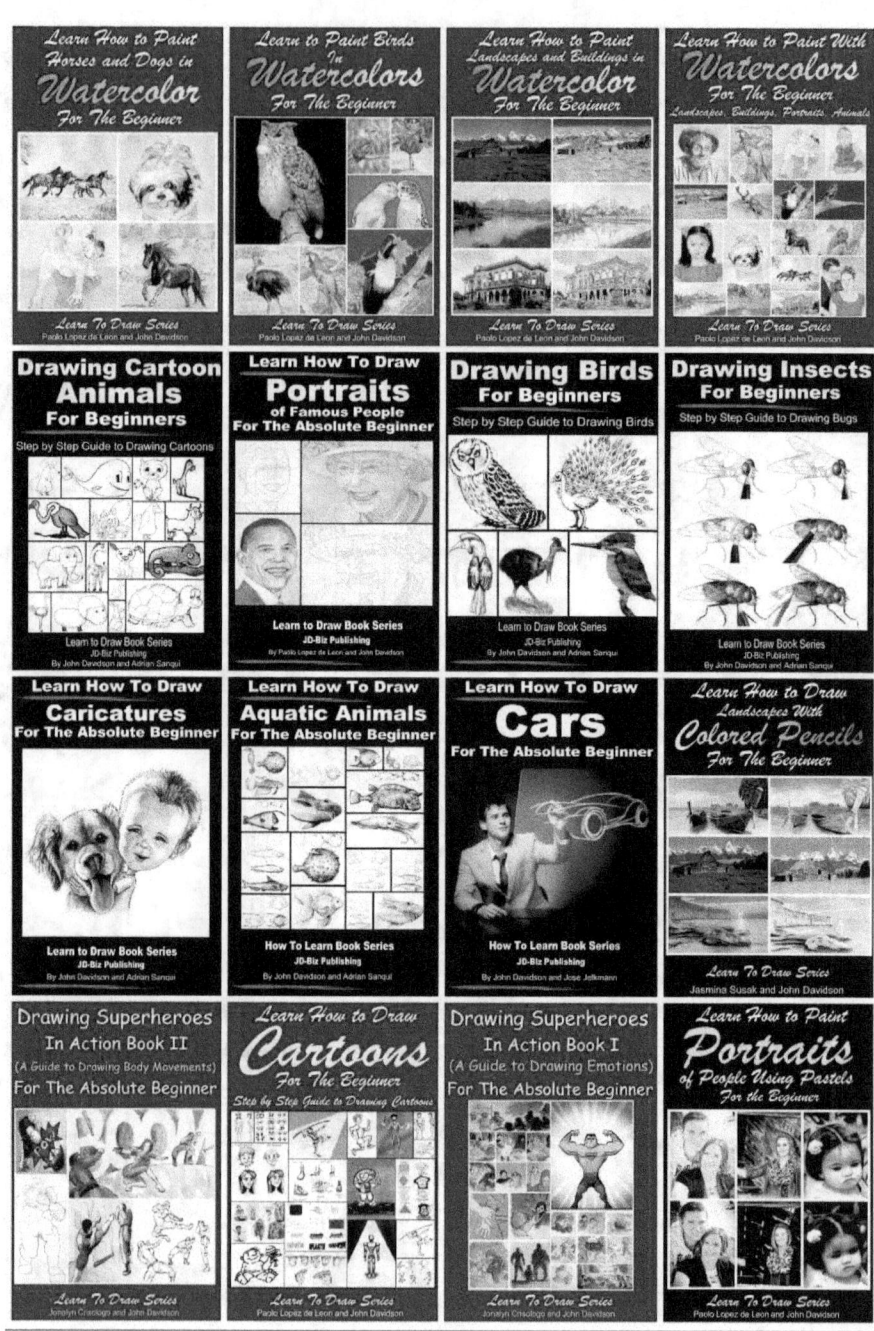

How to Build and Plan Books

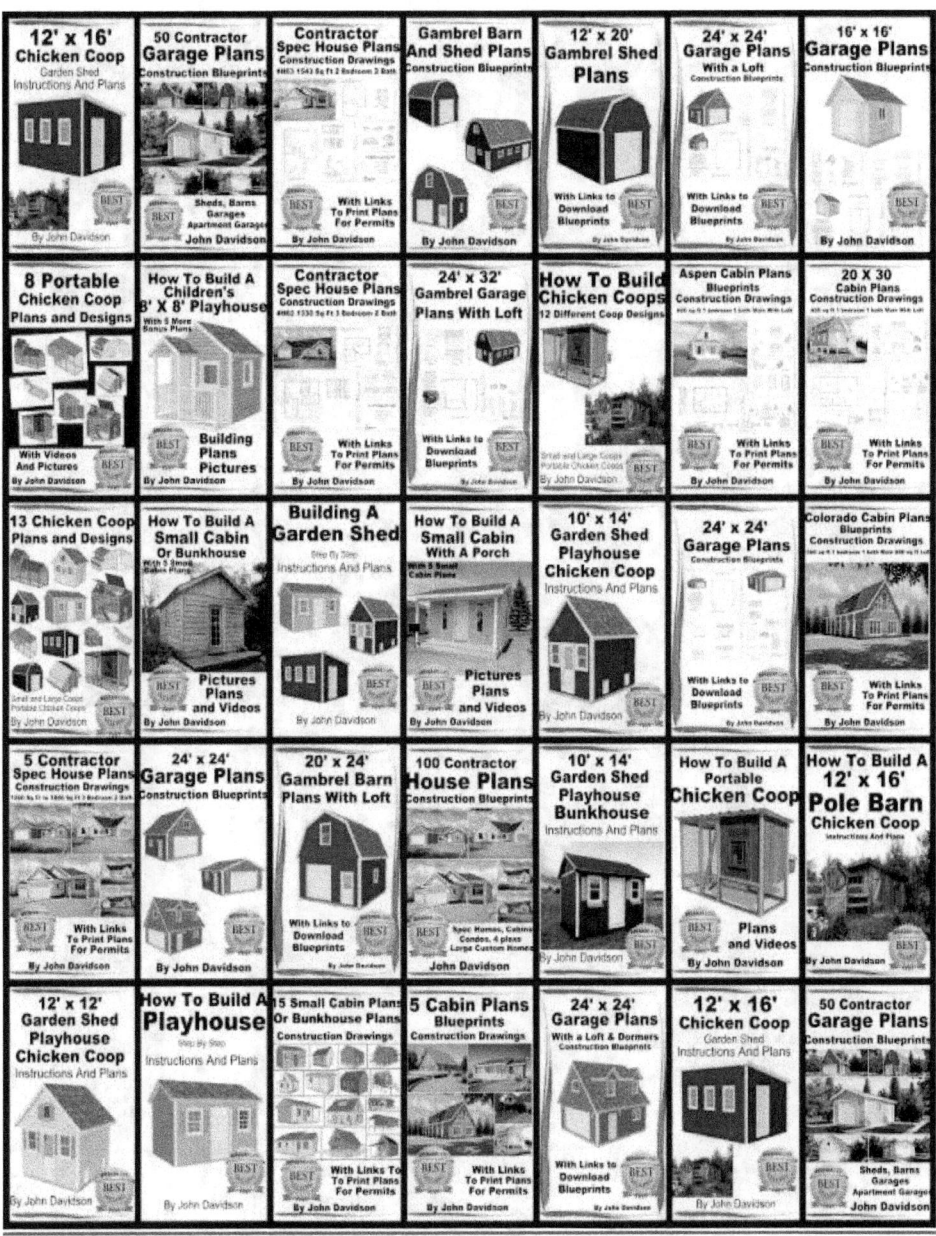

Entrepreneur Book Series

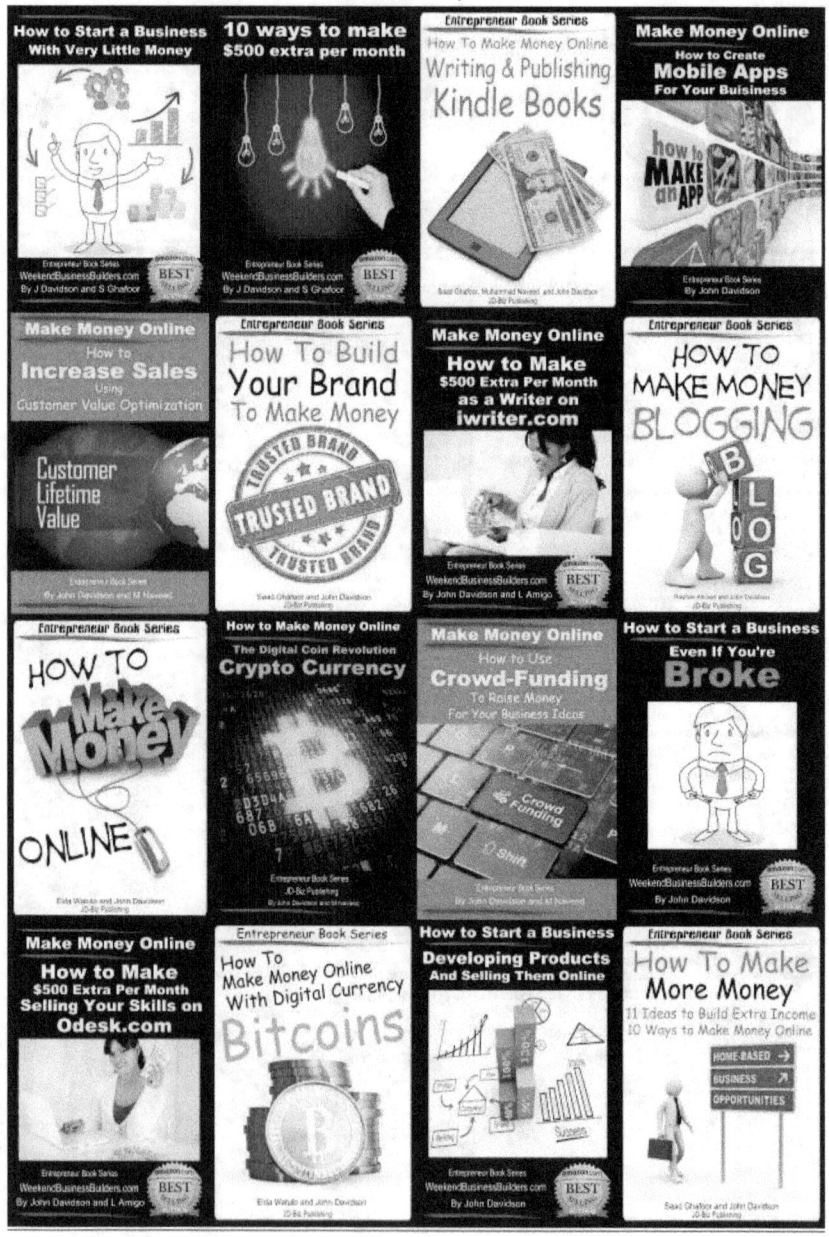

Publisher

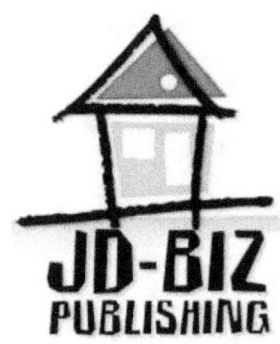

JD-Biz Corp

P O Box 374

Mendon, Utah 84325

http://www.jd-biz.com/

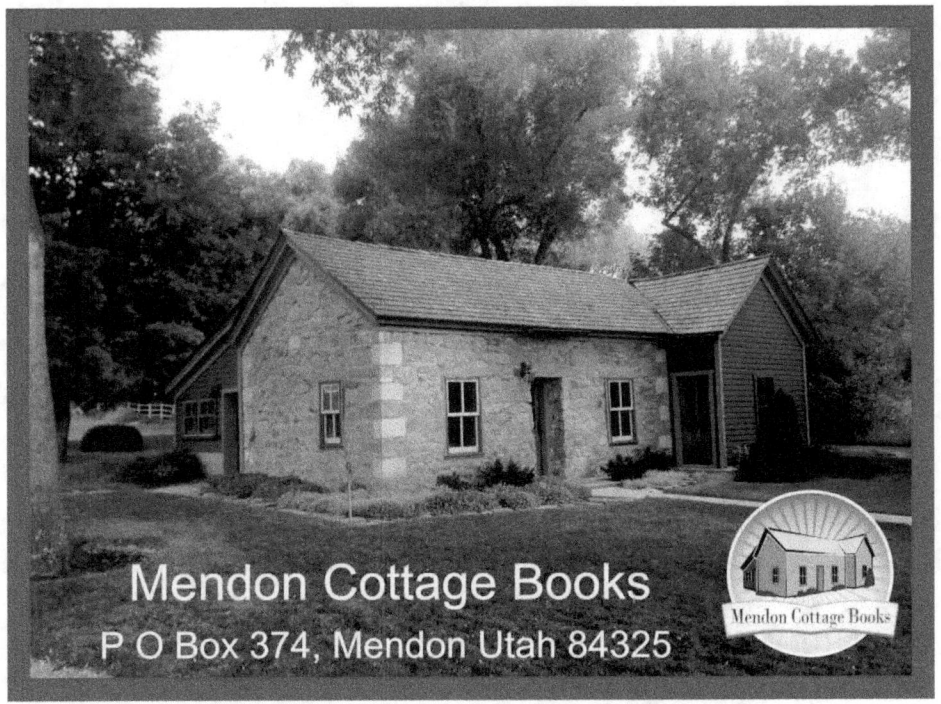

Mendon Cottage Books

P O Box 374, Mendon Utah 84325